FAST FACTS

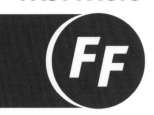

Indispensable
Guides to
Clinical
Practice

Erectile Dysfunction

Third edition

Culley Carson
Professor and Chief of Division of Urology,
The University of North Carolina,
Chapel Hill, North Carolina, USA

Simon Holmes
Consultant Urologist,
St Mary's Hospital, Portsmouth, UK

Roger S Kirby
Professor of Urology,
St George's Hospital, London, UK

With the compliments of

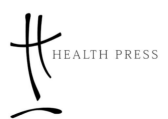
HEALTH PRESS

Oxford

Fast Facts – Erectile Dysfunction
First published as Fast Facts – Male Erectile Dysfunction 1997
Second edition 1998
Third edition September 2002

Text © 2002 Culley Carson, Simon Holmes, Roger S Kirby
© 2002 in this edition Health Press Limited
Health Press Limited, Elizabeth House, Queen Street,
Abingdon, Oxford OX14 3JR, UK
Tel: +44 (0)1235 523233
Fax: +44 (0)1235 523238

Fast Facts is a trade mark of Health Press Limited.

The publisher and the authors have made every effort to ensure the
accuracy of this book, but cannot accept responsibility for any errors
or omissions.

A CIP catalogue record for this title is available from the British Library.

ISBN 1-903734-05-3

Carson, C (Culley)
Fast Facts – Erectile Dysfunction/
Culley Carson, Simon Holmes, Roger S Kirby

Illustrated by Dee McLean, London, UK

Typeset by Zed, Oxford, UK

Printed by Fine Print (Services) Ltd, Oxford, UK

Glossary

cGMP: cyclic guanosine monophosphate, the second messenger molecule that facilitates the vasodilatation that leads to erection

Corpora cavernosa: paired columns of erectile tissue in the penis

Detumescence: loss of turgidity and erection, usually caused by active sympathetic stimulation

ED: erectile dysfunction

Intracavernosal self-injection: technique in which the patient injects vasoactive drugs into his own corpora cavernosa

MUSE®: medicated urethral system for erection

NO: nitric oxide, a neurotransmitter that produces an erection

Organic erectile dysfunction: erectile dysfunction caused by the failure of one or more of the essential stages in penile erection, namely the arterial blood supply, venous occlusion or neurological control

PDE 5: phosphodiesterase type 5, the substance that breaks down cGMP, resulting in detumescence

PGE$_1$: prostaglandin E$_1$, a neurotransmitter resulting in erection

Priapism: a persistent erection that lasts for more than 4 hours

Psychogenic erectile dysfunction: erectile dysfunction caused by higher brain centre influences in the presence of a normal erectile mechanism

Spinal erection centre: an area in the spinal cord through which the spinal erection reflex passes, and which is under neural control from higher brain centres

Tumescence: vasodilatation in the corpora cavernosa resulting in erection

Vasoactive agents: drugs that have a dilatory effect on blood vessels

VED: vacuum erection device

Veno-occlusive mechanism: the mechanism by which the venous drainage of the erectile tissues is occluded to allow filling of the lacunar spaces resulting in penile turgidity

VIP: vasoactive intestinal polypeptide – a neurotransmitter in the corpora cavernosa

Introduction

Just 25 years ago, male sexual health was considered to be the exclusive domain of the psychologist. Since then, surgeons have introduced penile prostheses and vacuum devices as mechanical treatments for erectile dysfunction (ED). More recently, basic scientists have determined the physiology of the erectile mechanism, leading to the development of a number of pharmacological treatment alternatives.

This progress has coincided with an increased understanding of the nature of male sexual health problems, and epidemiological data have confirmed that such problems are widely prevalent and the source of considerable morbidity, both for individuals and within relationships. ED is not a necessary part of the ageing process, but may occur as a result of a specific illness or as a consequence of the medical treatment of another unrelated illness. Healthcare professionals involved in all aspects of care need to be aware of these risks.

Patients now realize that simple, effective treatments are available and, increasingly, are demanding access to these therapies. The range of healthcare workers involved in the treatment of men with ED continues to expand with specialist nurses, nurse practitioners, primary care physicians and doctors from a variety of secondary care specialties expected to diagnose and treat patients and offer support and advice confidently and confidentially to these individuals. Therefore, it is essential that all healthcare professionals keep apace with developments to provide the best advice about the safety and effectiveness of treatment.

In response to these rapid advances in treatment, several sets of guidelines have been developed to help manage patients with ED. The guidelines include identification, assessment and diagnosis of the condition, modification of risk factors and provision of first- and second-line therapies. The third edition of *Fast Facts – Erectile Dysfunction* provides a more in-depth view of the overall management of ED and will be valuable to any healthcare professional who encounters men with the condition, particularly as the number of therapeutic options is increasing and patients expect to receive straightforward and effective treatment.

Epidemiology

Accurate figures for the prevalence of erectile dysfunction (ED) in male populations around the world are difficult to obtain. However, data from a number of US and UK studies are similar and these figures are regarded as the best estimate. The prevalence of complete ED is estimated to be approximately 5% among 40-year-olds, 10% among men in their 60s, 15% in their 70s and 30–40% in their 80s (Figure 1.1). From these figures it has been estimated that there may be 20 million men in the USA, and perhaps as many in Europe, who have significant problems with erectile function.

Risk factors for erectile dysfunction. Apart from age, other important risk factors for ED include diabetes mellitus, hypertension, hyperlipidaemia, depression and smoking (Table 1.1). Obesity, over-consumption of alcohol and lack of regular exercise may also contribute to the problem. Men with hypothyroidism and chronic renal

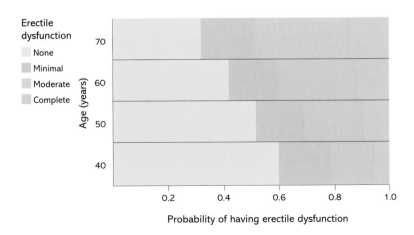

Probability of having erectile dysfunction

Figure 1.1 Relationship between age and the probability of erectile dysfunction. Data from the Massachusetts Male Aging Study, Feldman *et al. J Urol* 1994;150: 54–61.

TABLE 1.1

Prevalence of ED with specific medical conditions

Condition	Prevalence (%)
Overall (age 40–70 years)	10
Diabetes	35
Hypertension	25
Post MI	40
Severe depression	90
Cigarette smokers	20

failure are prone to ED, and hypogonadism and hyperprolactinaemia are also important causes of endocrine-associated erectile difficulties. Pelvic surgery may also result in ED.

Anatomy and physiology of the normal erection

The **penis** consists of three cylindrical columns of tissue surrounded by a sturdy fascial layer (Buck's fascia), subcutaneous tissue and skin

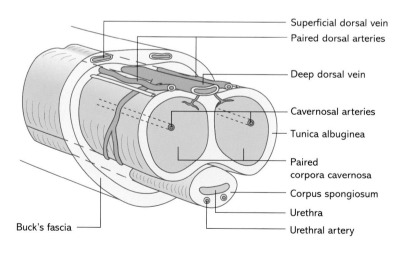

Superficial dorsal vein
Paired dorsal arteries
Deep dorsal vein
Cavernosal arteries
Tunica albuginea
Paired corpora cavernosa
Corpus spongiosum
Urethra
Urethral artery
Buck's fascia

Figure 1.2 Cross-sectional anatomy of the penis.

(Figure 1.2). Paired cylinders of erectile tissue, the corpora cavernosa, run the length of the penis, surrounded by a thick, non-expansile fibrous envelope, the tunica albuginea. Each corporal body communicates with the other through the medial septum that separates them. The erectile tissue itself is composed of a distensible lattice of blood sinusoids surrounded by trabeculae of smooth muscle, which control the sinusoidal blood capacity. The corpus spongiosum of the penis surrounds the urethra and expands to form the sensitive glans penis; it contains similar erectile tissue and is enclosed within the very thin tunica albuginea.

Vascular supply. The arterial blood flow to the penis (Figure 1.3) originates from the internal iliac arteries via the internal pudendal

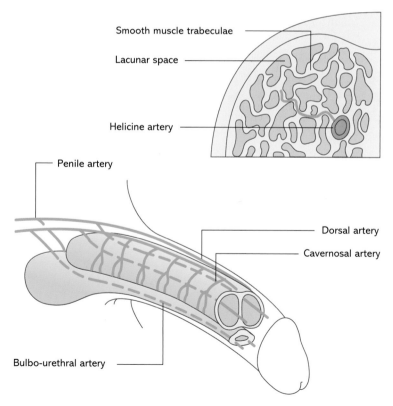

Smooth muscle trabeculae

Lacunar space

Helicine artery

Penile artery

Dorsal artery

Cavernosal artery

Bulbo-urethral artery

Figure 1.3 Arterial blood supply of the penis and corpora cavernosa.

arteries. The internal pudendal arteries terminate as the penile arteries, which divide to form:

- the dorsal artery
- the cavernosal artery, which runs down the centre of each corpus cavernosum
- the bulbo-urethral artery, which supplies the corpus spongiosum.

The cavernosal artery gives off numerous branches along its length, called helicine arteries, which supply blood to the sinusoids of the erectile tissue.

The venous drainage system collects blood from the sinusoids that run obliquely under the tunica albuginea, before exiting through the tunica as emissary veins to collect in the deep dorsal vein of the penis. The deep dorsal vein runs up the dorsal surface of the penis and joins the periprostatic venous complex (Figure 1.4). Cavernosal veins drain the proximal portions of the corpora.

Peripheral nerve supply. The mechanism of erection is controlled by the autonomic nervous system. Parasympathetic nerves from S2–4 are the principal mediators of erection, while sympathetic nerves from T11–L2 control ejaculation and detumescence. These autonomic fibres unite in the pelvic plexus to form the cavernous nerves, which run down behind the prostate and into the base of the penis. These nerves and the pelvic plexus itself are susceptible to damage from any form of pelvic surgery.

The pelvic nerves contain sensory and motor elements that form a reflex arc through the spinal cord, in an area known as the spinal erection centre. A 'reflex' erection therefore occurs as a direct result of stimulation of the penis, and can even occur in patients who have suffered a suprasacral spinal cord transection.

Mechanism of erection

Neuroendocrine messages from the brain (due to either audiovisual stimuli or fantasy), either with or without tactile stimulation of the penis, activate the autonomic nuclei of the spinal erection centre, which send messages to the erectile tissue of the corpora cavernosa via the cavernosal nerves. These result in:

- dilatation of the cavernosal and helicine arteries, increasing blood flow into the lacunar spaces
- relaxation of cavernosal smooth muscle, opening the vascular lacunar space
- expansion of the lacunar spaces against the tunica albuginea, compressing the obliquely running subtunical venous drainage channels, decreasing venous outflow and producing a rigid erection; this is the veno-occlusive mechanism (Figure 1.5).

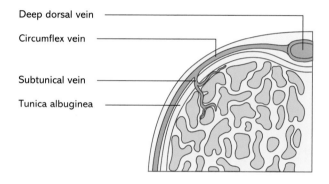

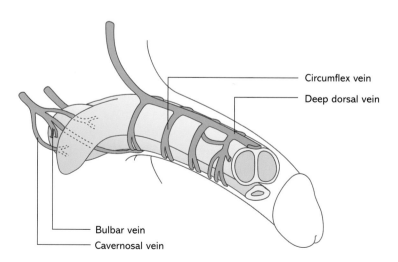

Figure 1.4 Venous drainage of the penis.

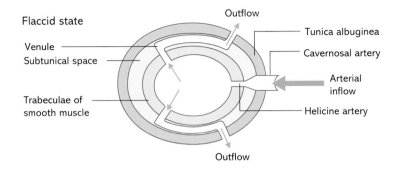

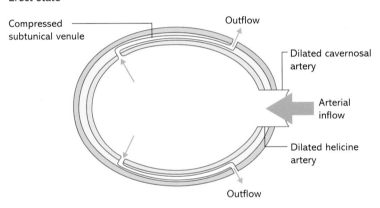

Figure 1.5 The veno-occlusive mechanism depends on compression of the subtunical venules.

Detumescence. Reversal of these events causes detumescence, and is caused by increased sympathetic vasoconstrictor activity and the enzymatic break- down of cyclic guanosine monophosphate (cGMP) by phosphodiesterase type 5 (PDE 5). This occurs naturally after orgasm and ejaculation, both of which are also mediated by the sympathetic nervous system.

Molecular basis of erection

The key modulator of erection is the tone of the smooth muscle walls of the helicine arteries and the trabecular spaces. This is controlled by the level of intracellular calcium in the smooth muscle cells. A number of neurotransmitters and endothelium-derived factors are able to influence intracellular calcium and thereby alter the balance between penile flaccidity and erection (Figure 1.6).

Smooth-muscle relaxation. Nitric oxide (NO) is the most important neurotransmitter in this system. Produced from L-arginine by the enzyme nitric oxide synthase, NO diffuses into the smooth muscle cells, where it activates a guanylate cyclase second messenger system. Guanylate cyclase converts guanosine triphosphate (GTP) into cGMP. This then activates the sodium pump system and opens potassium channels, causing a decrease in intracellular calcium. The effect of cGMP is ended by enzymatic breakdown; the enzyme involved, PDE 5, exists principally in the corpora cavernosa.

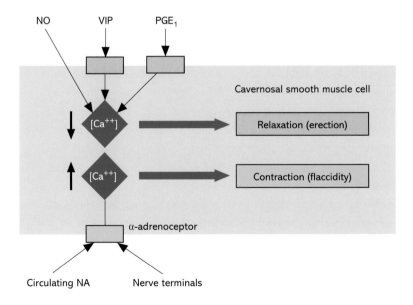

Figure 1.6 Factors that influence balance between erection and flaccidity. NA, noradrenaline; NO, nitric oxide; PGE_1, prostaglandin E_1; VIP, vasoactive intestinal polypeptide.

Other vasodilator mechanisms exist, including ones involving vasoactive intestinal polypeptide (VIP) and prostaglandin E_1 (PGE_1), both of which act through the adenylate cyclase system. VIP and PGE_1 molecules stimulate the production of cyclic adenosine monophosphate (cAMP) from adenosine triphosphate (ATP). Like cGMP, cAMP reduces intracellular calcium and thereby induces smooth-muscle relaxation.

Smooth-muscle contraction. The vasoconstrictor noradrenaline (NA) counterbalances the smooth-muscle relaxation mechanisms. Noradrenaline is released from sympathetic nerve terminals within the corpora, and diffuses across the synaptic gap. It activates α_1-adrenoceptors on the cell membranes of smooth muscle cells. These α_1-adrenoceptors are linked to second messenger pathways that raise intracellular calcium, either by facilitating entry of calcium from the extracellular compartment, or by releasing calcium from intracellular organelles. A number of other molecules that increase intracellular calcium, such as endothelin-1 and prostaglandin F_2, are also involved in the maintenance of flaccidity. Increased free calcium levels within the smooth muscle cells of the helicine arteries and the trabecular smooth muscle cells activate the contractile mechanism by which actin and myosin molecules slide over each other and form new cross bridges. Once these are created, a tonic contractile state can be maintained with almost zero energy consumption.

Neural influence

A number of neural pathways to and from the brain influence and sometimes initiate an erectile response. A 'psychogenic' erection occurs as a result of audiovisual stimuli, erotic thoughts or sexual fantasy via signals from the brain to the spinal erection centre activating the erectile process (Figure 1.7). However, these pathways can also act to inhibit the same process, giving rise to psychogenic ED. Several areas in the brain are important in this respect. One is the paraventricular nucleus of the hypothalamus, where dopamine is the key neurotransmitter mediating coordination of neuronal activity.

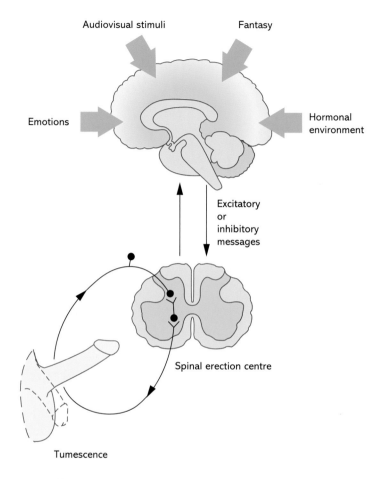

Figure 1.7 Neural pathways that influence the erectile response.

Causes of erectile dysfunction

The causes of ED (Table 1.2) may be due to changes in the:

- CNS, at the level of either the brain or the spinal cord
- peripheral nervous system, usually due to diabetes mellitus, trauma or surgical injury
- corpora cavernosa, as in Peyronie's disease
- vascular system – either arterial insufficiency or a disorder of the veno-occlusive mechanism
- endocrine system – reduced testosterone or increased prolactin.

15

TABLE 1.2

Causes of erectile dysfunction

Psychogenic

- Anxiety
- Loss of attraction
- Relationship difficulties
- Stress

Psychiatric

- Depression

Neurogenic

- Trauma
- Myelodysplasia (spina bifida)
- Intervertebral disc lesion
- Multiple sclerosis
- Diabetes mellitus
- Alcohol
- Pelvic surgery
- Pelvic radiotherapy

Endocrine

- Hormonal deficiency – low testosterone; raised sex-hormone-binding globulin; high prolactin

Arteriogenic

- Hypertension
- Smoking
- Diabetes mellitus
- Hyperlipidaemia
- Peripheral vascular disease

Venous

- Functional impairment of the veno-occlusive mechanism

Drugs

- Central and/or direct effect, most commonly implicated antihypertensives, antidepressants and luteinizing hormone-releasing hormone analogues

These conditions are not mutually exclusive; many cases of erectile dysfunction are multifactorial

Although it was originally believed that psychogenic problems were the predominant cause of ED, it has now been shown that organic causes are very common, particularly in middle-aged and older men presenting to an ED clinic. In one study, for example, 11% of new patients attending an ED clinic were found to have undiagnosed diabetes and more than half had vascular problems. Almost all patients, however, have some psychogenic component to their symptoms, often caused by anxiety and loss of confidence.

Epidemiology and pathophysiology – Key points

- Approximately 10% of men between 40 and 70 years of age have moderate or severe ED.
- Patients with certain medical conditions have an increased risk of ED, and erectile difficulties should be actively sought.
- Multiple neurotransmitters are involved in the mechanism of erectile function – nitric oxide is probably the most important.
- An erection is a vascular event under neurological control.

Key references

Fedele D, Coscelli C, Santeusanio F et al. Erectile dysfunction in diabetic subjects in Italy. Gruppo Italiano Studio Deficit Erettile nei Diabetici. *Diabetes Care* 1998;21:1973–7.

Feldman HA, Goldstein I, Hatzichristou DG et al. Impotence and its medical and psychological correlates: results of the Massachusetts Male Aging Study. *J Urol* 1994;150:54–61.

Fournier GR, Juenemann KP, Lue TF, Tanagho EA. Mechanism of venous occlusion during canine penile erection. An anatomical demon-stration. *J Urol* 1987;137:163–7.

Johannes CB, Araujo AB, Feldman HA et al. Incidence of erectile dysfunction in men 40 to 69 years old. Longitudinal results from the Massachusetts Male Aging Study. *J Urol* 2000;163:460–3.

Kinsey AC, Pomeroy W, Martin C. Age and sexual outlet. In: Kinsey AC, Pomeroy W, Martin C, eds. *Sexual Behaviour in the Human Male.* Philadelphia: WB Saunders, 1948:218–62.

Lerner SE, Melman A, Christ GJ. A review of erectile dysfunction: new insights and more questions. *J Urol* 1993;149:1246–55.

Lue TF, Tanagho EA. Functional anatomy and mechanism of penile erection. In: Lue TF, Tanagho EA, McClure RD, eds. *Contemporary Management of Impotence and Infertility.* Baltimore: Williams and Wilkins, 1988:39–50.

NIH Consensus Development Panel on Impotence. *JAMA* 1993;270: 83–90.

Wagner G, Saenz de Tejada I. Update on male erectile dysfunction. *BMJ* 1998; 316:678–82.

Walsh PC, Mostwin JL. Radical prostatectomy and cystoprostatectomy with preservation of potency: results using a new nerve-sparing technique. *Br J Urol* 1984;56:694–7.

A full history and thorough clinical examination of the patient are needed to:
- help elucidate the cause of ED
- determine whether the problem is psychogenic or organic in origin
- identify any clinical signs of the known risk factors.

It should be borne in mind that ED can be an early symptom of a significant systemic condition, such as diabetes mellitus or vascular disease.

Referral to an appropriate physician may be necessary if there is evidence of:
- significant peripheral vascular or cardiac disease
- an organic cause of ED in a young man (e.g. depression)
- hypogonadism in a young man.

Findings from the history and examination of the patient can be supplemented by investigations to identify the cause of erectile failure. Investigations can be used to:
- confirm the associated underlying condition (e.g. diabetes mellitus)
- give a differential diagnosis of specific causes of ED.

History

A detailed history is probably the most important aspect of the patient assessment. The clinical history has several purposes:
- to confirm that the patient is suffering from ED
- to assess the severity of the condition
- to identify a possible underlying aetiology
- to assess the fitness of the patient for resuming sexual activity.

The initial aim, therefore, is to determine whether the problem is one of ED and whether or not this is accompanied by ejaculatory dysfunction, diminished libido or loss of orgasm.

The terminology associated with ED is often confused, and men's expectations of their sexual function may be unrealistic. The severity of the problem can often be assessed by asking simple questions (Table 2.1).

TABLE 2.1

Suitable initial questions to ask the patient with ED

- What is the problem with your erections?
- How frequently do you have the problem?
- When did you last have successful sexual intercourse?
- How strong is your desire for sex, now and in the past?
- What has been the effect of your sexual difficulties on your relationship with your partner?
- What is your partner's attitude towards the problem?
- What are you and your partner hoping to gain from any treatments that may be available?

Many doctor/patient consultations about ED are initiated by the doctor. The patient may present with an unrelated problem and only when questioned more closely will he reveal his true concerns. Likewise, there are a number of medical conditions that are now well recognized as being associated with ED (Table 1.1 on page 8). Many patients are relieved, indeed pleased, to discuss the problem once the issue has been raised.

Once the degree of ED has been established, tactful enquiries can be made about a possible aetiology. The aim of the subsequent discussion is to differentiate between obvious psychological causes and organic causes of the problem. Many men have a combination of causes, however, and the history will contain both organic and psychogenic elements. Topics to cover in discussions with patients include:

- the patient's sexual development and the onset of the problem
- the patient's and his partner's attitude to the problem
- the presence of any obvious stress factors, such as marital problems, financial concerns, sexual inhibitions
- medical and drug history, in particular smoking, chronic medical illness, pelvic, perineal or penile surgery, pelvic radiotherapy, recreational drug use or psychiatric illness.

The diagnosis of psychogenic and/or organic causes is based on a number of factors.

Psychogenic erectile dysfunction. The association between anxiety and ED should be established. A psychological element should be suspected in a patient who obtains an erection during foreplay or self-stimulation, but fails or fears failure on penetration. Performance anxiety is almost universal in men with a purely psychogenic problem. In these men, early morning and nocturnal erections are often preserved (Table 2.2). Onset of dysfunction is usually sudden and may relate to a specific occasion or life event. A more detailed psychosexual history, exploring sources of anxiety, guilt, relationship difficulties or depression should be obtained.

Organic erectile dysfunction is characterized by a progressive loss of erectile function with a gradual loss of sustainable erectile rigidity, often combined with the loss of early morning and nocturnal erections (Table 2.2). Both libido and ejaculatory function are usually maintained. Several systems have been developed to score the erectile problem objectively. The International Index of Erectile Function (IIEF) has been widely used to quantify the problem. However, the recent International Consultation on Erectile Dysfunction has recommended a variation of this system that is slightly easier to use and is expected to gain favour (Table 2.3). The scoring system provides a method of measuring a patient's progress from an initial 'benchmark' level.

TABLE 2.2

Differential diagnosis of psychogenic and organic ED

Psychogenic	Organic
• Sudden onset	• Gradual onset
• Specific situation	• All circumstances
• Normal nocturnal and early morning erections	• Absent nocturnal and early morning erections
• Relationship problems	• Normal libido and ejaculation
• Problems during sexual development	• Normal sexual development

TABLE 2.3

ED intensity scale

Each question has several responses. Circle the number of the response that best describes your own situation. Please be sure that you select one and only one response for each question.

1. How often were you able to get an erection during sexual activity?	Almost never or never	A few times (much less than half the time)
	1	2
2. When you had erections with sexual stimulation, how often were your erections hard enough for penetration (entering your partner)?	Almost never or never	A few times (much less than half the time)
	1	2
3. When you attempted intercourse, how often were you able to penetrate (enter) your partner?	Almost never or never	A few times (much less than half the time)
	1	2
4. During sexual intercourse, how often were you able to maintain your erection after you had penetrated (entered) your partner?	Almost never or never	A few times (much less than half the time)
	1	2
5. During sexual intercourse, how difficult was it to maintain your erection to completion of intercourse?	Extremely difficult	Very difficult
	1	2

Instructions for scoring: Add the scores for each item 1–5 (total possible score = 25). ED Severity Classification: Total score 5–10 (severe); 11–15 (moderate); 16–20 (mild); 21–25 (normal). Adapted from Cappelleri et al., Urology 1999;54:346–51.

Concomitant medication. A detailed medical history should be taken to check for the presence of any recognized risk factors. In particular, careful enquiry should be made about current medications, as well as the use of recreational drugs. A number of these may cause or contribute to ED (Table 2.4). For example, antihypertensive agents, such as β-blockers and diuretics, are associated with ED. In such cases it may be worthwhile changing the patient's medication to an α-adrenoceptor

Sometimes (about half the time)	Most times (much more than half the time)	Almost always or always
3	4	5
Sometimes (about half the time)	Most times (much more than half the time)	Almost always or always
3	4	5
Sometimes (about half the time)	Most times (much more than half the time)	Almost always or always
3	4	5
Sometimes (about half the time)	Most times (much more than half the time)	Almost always or always
3	4	5
Difficult	Slightly difficult	Not difficult
3	4	5

antagonist such as doxazosin or terazosin. Because of the vasodilatory effects of this class of drug, they may be mildly beneficial in ED, particularly in combination with a phosphodiesterase type 5 inhibitor.

Erectile dysfunction is a common complication of antidepressant therapy with either monoamine oxidase inhibitors or tricyclic antidepressants. Selective serotonin re-uptake inhibitors may cause both ED and retarded ejaculation.

Physical examination

The examination of a man with ED will be directed, to a certain extent, by knowledge gained from his history. However, it is important to assess the external genitalia, the endocrine and vascular systems, and the prostate gland in most patients (Figure 2.1).

The presence, location and size of the testes, together with an assessment of secondary sexual characteristics, will usually be enough to identify obvious hypogonadism.

Vascular assessment should include measurement of blood pressure, cardiac status and lower extremity pulses; a palpable aortic aneurysm should be sought. The penis should be carefully palpated to exclude the presence of fibrous Peyronie's plaques and to check for phimosis.

The prostate should be the same rubbery consistency as the tip of the nose. The presence of induration, or a palpable nodule, should raise the

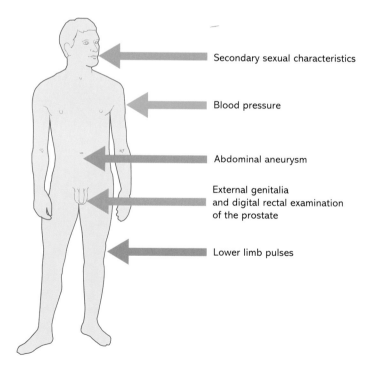

Secondary sexual characteristics

Blood pressure

Abdominal aneurysm

External genitalia
and digital rectal examination
of the prostate

Lower limb pulses

Figure 2.1 Important aspects of the physical examination in men with erectile dysfunction.

TABLE 2.4

Medications associated with ED

Major tranquilizers

- Phenothiazines
  (e.g. fluphenazine,
  chlorpromazine, promazine,
  mesoridazine)
- Butyrophenones
  (e.g. haloperidol)
- Thioxanthines (e.g. thiothixene,
  chlorprothixene)

Anticholinergics

- Atropine
- Propantheline
- Dimenhydrinate
- Diphenhydramine

Luteinizing hormone-releasing hormone analogues

Antiandrogens

Antihypertensives

- Diuretics (e.g. thiazides,
  spironolactone)
- Vasodilators (e.g. hydralazine)
- Central sympatholytics
  (e.g. methyldopa, clonidine,
  reserpine)
- Ganglion blockers (e.g.
  guanethidine, bethanidine)
- β-blockers (e.g. propranolol,
  metoprolol, atenolol)
- ACE inhibitors (e.g. enalapril)
- Calcium channel blockers
  (e.g. nifedipine)

Antidepressants

- Tricyclics (e.g. nortriptyline,
  amitriptyline, desipramine,
  doxepin)
- Monoamine oxidase inhibitors
  (e.g. isocarboazide, phenelzine,
  tranylcypromine, pargyline,
  procarbine)

Anxiolytics

- Benzodiazepines
  (e.g. chlordiazepoxide,
  diazepam, clorazepate)

Psychotropic drugs

- Alcohol
- Marijuana
- Amphetamines
- Barbiturates
- Nicotine
- Opiates

Miscellaneous

- Cimetidine
- Clofibrate
- Digoxin
- Oestrogens
- Indomethacin
- Many others

suspicion of prostate cancer. Serum levels of prostate-specific antigen (PSA) should be obtained and, if they are elevated in relation to the patient's age and a diagnosis of prostate cancer is likely to be of clinical value, he should be referred for transrectal ultrasound (TRUS)-guided biopsy.

Clinical investigations

The degree to which men should undergo clinical investigation depends on the history of the problem, the experience of the physician and the preferences of the patient. There have been several clinical guidelines published regarding the management of men with ED. Most concur that the investigations performed on each patient should address his particular complaints. The investigations can be divided into essential, possible and specialized (Table 2.5). Diabetes mellitus should be excluded by testing the urine and blood for excess glucose; this is the only essential investigation. In some circumstances, treatment may then be initiated without further investigation. If this treatment is not successful, referral for specialist advice will probably be required.

TABLE 2.5

Clinical investigations for ED

Essential	Possible	Specialized
• Urine dipstick	• Serum testosterone	• Nocturnal penile tumescence testing
• Serum glucose	• Sex-hormone-binding globulin	• Colour Doppler imaging
	• Prolactin	• Pharmaco-cavernosography
	• Creatinine	• Pharmaco-arteriography
	• Thyroid hormones	• Psychiatric evaluation
	• Fasting lipid profile	• Vascular evaluation
	• Prostate-specific antigen	• Cardiac evaluation
	• Follicle-stimulating hormone/luteinizing hormone	

General investigations include serum concentrations of testosterone, sex-hormone-binding globulin (SHBG), prolactin, creatinine, thyroid hormones, PSA and fasting lipid levels (Table 2.6). Special investigations are not always required, but may be necessary if patients fail to respond to minimally invasive treatments before other options can be explored. Unless the problem is obviously psychogenic, a proportion of patients will have a trial injection of an intracavernosal vasoactive agent (see page 48) and their response assessed.

Specialized investigations need only be performed when a detailed knowledge of the cause of ED is required, and the patient and his partner have expressed an interest in pursuing corrective therapy or if there is concern about a patient resuming sexual activity. A specialist referral is usually required (Table 2.7).

Nocturnal penile tumescence testing. The presence of nocturnal erections, which is used to differentiate psychogenic from organic impotence, can be detected using devices placed around the penis during sleep. This is known as nocturnal penile tumescence (NPT) testing. The Snap-Gauge band and RigiScan device are designed to be used at home and record the occurrence of nocturnal erections. Determining the presence or absence of nocturnal erections can also help treatment decisions.

TABLE 2.6

Investigations to identify underlying physiological conditions associated with ED

Investigation	Indication
Prolactin	Low testosterone
PSA	Prostatic symptoms or suspicion of prostate cancer
Creatinine	Suspicion of renal impairment
Thyroid hormones	Suspicion of thyroid disease
Liver function tests	Suspicion of liver disease
Lipid profile	Suspicion of peripheral vascular disease

TABLE 2.7

Specific indications for referral to a specialist

- Patient request for specific testing
- Patient requiring vascular, neurological or cardiac evaluation
- Young patient, severe problem
- Patient with Peyronie's disease
- Patient with refractory depression, psychosis or complex psychosexual disorder
- Patients who fail initial therapy

Colour Doppler imaging provides information about penile haemo-dynamics after maximal smooth-muscle relaxation has been induced with a vasoactive agent. Its aim is to distinguish arterial insufficiency from other causes of erectile failure.

Pharmacocavernosography. Failure of the veno-occlusive mechanism to provide adequate venous outflow resistance can be demonstrated by pharmacocavernosography. This measures the blood flow required to maintain a pharmacologically stimulated erection. Contrast medium injected into the corpora will identify the location of any leak, which often originates in the deep dorsal vein of the penis (Figure 2.2), but may also be present in less accessible cavernosal veins.

Pharmaco-arteriography. In young men with ED caused by pelvic or perineal trauma, pudendal arteriography before and after a

Diagnosis – Key points

- ED is a good index of overall male health. It is associated with vascular disease, smoking, diabetes, depression and other conditions. It is the responsibility of the clinician to seek out a possible cause.
- The patient's history is perhaps the most important diagnostic tool.
- Patient investigations are tailored to the history, examination and suspected cause of ED.

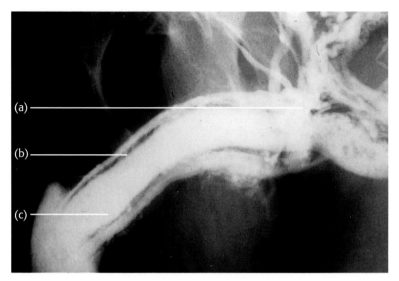

Figure 2.2 Venous leakage is occurring through the dorsal vein and into the retropubic venous plexus during pharmacocavernosography: (a) retropubic venous plexus; (b) dorsal vein; (c) corpus cavernosum.

pharmacologically stimulated erection may identify those requiring arterial bypass.

Key references

Cappelleri JC, Rosen RC, Smith MD et al. Diagnostic evaluation of the erectile function domain of the International Index of Erectile Function. *Urology* 1999;54:346–57.

Kirby RS. Impotence: diagnosis and management of erectile dysfunction. *BMJ* 1994;308:957–61.

Krane RJ. Medical progress. Impotence. *N Engl J Med* 1989;321:1648–58.

Process of Care Panel. Position Paper: The process of care model for evaluation and treatment of erectile dysfunction. *Int J Impot Res* 1999;11:59–74.

Rosen RC, Riley A, Wagner G et al. The International Index of Erectile Function (IIEF): a multidimensional scale for the assessment of erectile dysfunction. *Urology* 1997;49: 822–30.

The treatment options for psychogenic and organic ED depend on the experience of the clinician, the wishes of the patient and the facilities that are available (Table 3.1). An approach to the treatment and management of ED is summarized in Figure 3.1.

Modification of risk factors

Some patients will have recognized risk factors for the onset of ED. Primary advice should be aimed at reversing these adverse factors. For example, cigarette smoking or the use of recreational drugs should be discouraged, and depression or dyslipidaemia recognized and addressed. If the onset of ED is associated with the introduction of a new therapeutic drug (such as an antihypertensive), then an alternative agent should be sought. These lifestyle changes should be recommended, whatever the cause of the ED, as erectile function can be an indicator of general well-being.

Psychogenic erectile dysfunction

Erections are often stimulated by audiovisual stimuli or fantasy; in the same way, however, other CNS signals can inhibit the erectile response.

TABLE 3.1

Treatment options in psychogenic and organic ED

Psychogenic	Organic
• Psychosexual therapy	• Oral pharmacological agents
• Oral pharmacological agents	• Intraurethral therapy
• Intraurethral therapy	• Intracavernosal therapy
• Intracavernosal therapy	• Vacuum devices
	• Androgen replacement therapy
	• Surgery

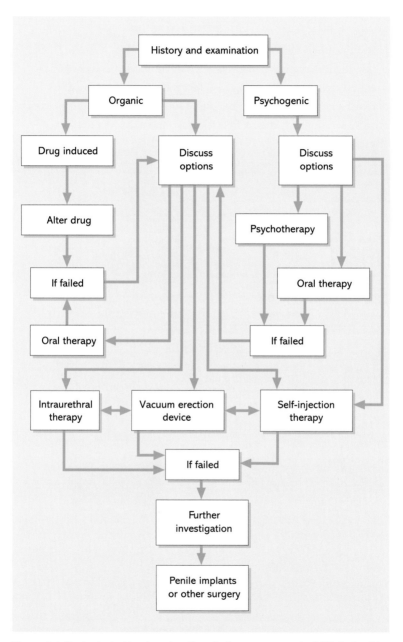

Figure 3.1 Goal-oriented treatment options in the management of ED. It should be remembered that, at any stage, the patient may decide to opt out of therapy and simply accept his condition.

Inhibitory messages from the brain, acting on the spinal erection centre, prevent not only the 'psychogenic' erection, but also the 'reflex' erection by modulating the normal reflex arc. The inhibitory influence of the brain on erectile function may also be caused by an increased sympathetic outflow and the release of systemic catecholamines, which are known to inhibit the erectile response and cause detumescence (Figure 3.2).

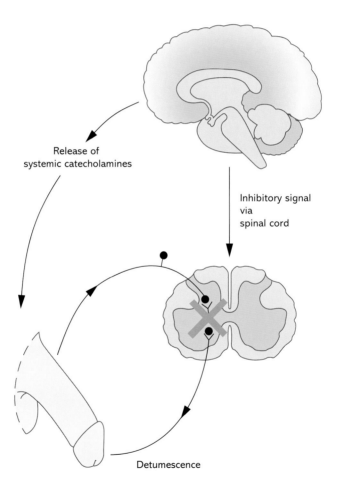

Release of
systemic catecholamines

Inhibitory signal
via
spinal cord

Detumescence

Figure 3.2 The inhibitory influence of the brain on erectile function via the sympathetic nervous system.

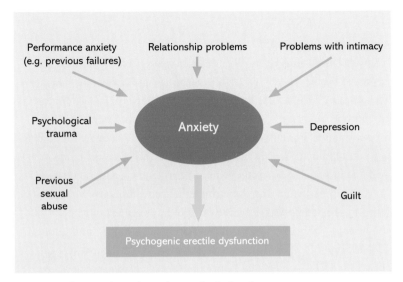

Figure 3.3 Causes of psychogenic erectile dysfunction.

Psychogenic ED can be caused by a number of problems, such as performance anxiety, guilt, depression, relationship problems, or by fear and personal anxiety (Figure 3.3). Performance anxiety is a particularly common cause of erectile problems and may be self-perpetuating, with any subsequent attempts at sexual contact being burdened by a 'fear of failure' that only serves to exacerbate the problem. Concerns over whether an adequate and sustainable erection will develop, lead to 'spectatoring' (i.e. anxious scrutiny of a developing erection), which only serves to inhibit normal sexual responses further.

Treatment alternatives in this situation are either:

- to identify the source of anxiety, guilt or depression and provide a psychological treatment
- to initiate a physical (drug) treatment that overcomes the specific problem of ED.

Once a patient can obtain an erection 'on demand' from a physical therapy, he may overcome performance anxiety himself.

Psychosexual therapy. Treatment for psychogenic ED cannot be standardized because the source of anxiety varies between patients. Relationship difficulties, depression, guilt, problems with intimacy and

33

lack of sexual experience may all increase anxiety and/or conflict that may be manifested as ED.

Psychosexual treatments range from simple sex education through improved partner communication to cognitive and behavioural therapy. The onus is on the counsellor to identify the source of anxiety and select an appropriate therapy. Sex education usually involves correction of misinformation and ignorance about normal sexual practice. Improving partner communication may allow partners to overcome their embarrassment about sexual matters and express their sexual needs and desires.

Modern sex therapy owes much to the contribution of Masters and Johnson. They described a treatment programme involving a combination of behavioural and psychosexual elements, and reported a 70% success rate after 5 years of follow up. Today, therapy is more behaviour-based and aims to reduce performance anxiety via a programmed relearning of a couple's sexual behaviour. Often, this is achieved by gradually increasing a couple's repertoire of sexual activities that do not depend on maintaining a full erection, until full confidence is restored.

The drawback to these types of therapy is that they are expensive in terms of time and resources. They also usually require the presence and co-operation of the sexual partner, though initial individual consultations often help identify relationship problems and expectations. Few long-term studies have assessed the eventual outcomes of these treatments, though there appears to be a substantial recurrence rate after therapy. Many couples, however, derive genuine benefit from this approach, which can also be usefully combined with oral pharmacological therapy.

Physical therapies

Oral pharmacological agents. Although oral drug therapies have historically had a very limited role in the treatment of men with ED, it is now apparent that well-tolerated and successful treatment is possible. It is believed that most patients suffering from ED will respond to pharmacological agents in the not so distant future.

The 'on-demand' concept is the basis of other physical treatments such as intracavernosal and intraurethral drugs, and vacuum devices.

However, the rates of discontinuation with these treatment alternatives are high due to side-effects, dislike of needles and unwillingness of the partner to participate. This has provided the stimulus for the development of effective oral drugs – many are under development, awaiting approval or have recently been released. Because many of these agents have different sites of action, it is anticipated that drug combinations act synergistically, though at present this remains a hypothesis rather than a proven fact.

Intraurethral therapy. These treatments deliver vasoactive drugs to the corpora cavernosa via the urethral mucosa. The urethra has a rich submucosal blood supply that communicates with the corpora cavernosa through the corpus spongiosum, allowing delivery of vasoactive drugs to the corporal bodies. Therapeutic drug levels can be achieved in men with both psychogenic and organic ED.

Intracavernosal therapy. Erections can be stimulated pharmacologically using a vasoactive drug; this can be used to treat psychogenic ED enabling intercourse to take place and, with time, may eradicate the 'fear of failure' anxiety associated with the condition. Reliance on the drug to produce a satisfactory erection should then diminish, until eventually it is no longer required.

Combined psychogenic/organic erectile dysfunction

A large proportion of patients have a combination of psychogenic and organic ED. Erectile failure resulting from a developing organic problem may provoke the onset of a psychogenic effect once the patient develops the 'fear of failure' on sexual contact. To treat these men holistically, the family physician and psychotherapist may need to collaborate and combine counselling with a physical therapy, such as an oral pharmacological agent.

Organic erectile dysfunction

Organic ED will only respond to physical therapy. Treatment can be either cause-specific and aim to correct an identifiable abnormality, or general and aim to provide an erectile response regardless of underlying cause. The appropriate treatment option will vary according to the patient's cultural, religious and economic status. Consider:

- ease of administration
- invasiveness
- reversibility
- cost
- mechanism of action
- side effects.

Androgen replacement therapy. Male hypogonadism, leading to testosterone deficiency and impotence, can have a number of causes (Table 3.2). Regardless of aetiology, the aim of androgen replacement therapy is to maintain secondary sexual characteristics and sexual behaviour. Although erectile function can be improved or restored in men with marked androgen deficiency, it is less clear whether men with borderline levels obtain any great benefit from testosterone supplementation. It is known that serum testosterone levels, sexual desire and erectile function all diminish with age, but it is less clear whether testosterone replacement will necessarily result in improved erections. The precise role of testosterone in erectile function remains

TABLE 3.2

Causes of hypogonadism

Hypogonadotrophic (hypothalamic–pituitary dysfunction)

- Drugs, e.g. luteinizing hormone-releasing hormone analogues
- Pituitary tumour
- Congenital: Kallmann's syndrome
- Prader–Willi syndrome
- Bilateral orchidectomy

Hypergonadotrophic (primary testicular failure)

- Gonadal dysgenesis
- Rudimentary testis syndrome
- Congenital: Klinefelter's syndrome

> **Treatment options – Key points**
>
> - Modification of risk factors should be recommended (as advice on overall male health) but rarely leads to restoration of sexual function.
> - Partner communication is an important aspect of sexual function and therefore dysfunction.
> - Psychogenic ED results from a multitude of relationship problems and anxieties.

controversial. For example, around 20% of men undergoing androgen deprivation to treat prostate cancer retain erections sufficient for sexual intercourse. Androgens are known to support both CNS and corpus cavernosum function, with both libido and smooth-muscle relaxation facilitated by testosterone. All hormone substitution therapy aims to achieve physiological serum concentrations of both the hormone and its active metabolites, but current androgen replacement therapies do not always achieve this. Testosterone replacement can be administered orally, by intramuscular injection, via skin patches or gel. Patches are applied to either the back, abdomen, upper arms or thighs (Andropatch™ or Virormone™) or the scrotum (Testoderm™). Skin reactivity may develop in a proportion of patients. A new 1% testosterone gel (Androgel™) has been approved for use in the USA. A daily application enhances serum testosterone levels and has minimal dermatological side-effects.

All forms of androgen replacement carry the theoretical risk of stimulating prostate growth and promoting the development of latent foci of prostate cancer. Although it is difficult to quantify these risks, and they are probably small, it is important that any patient receiving this treatment is fully informed and has his prostate-specific antigen (PSA) level monitored. Other side-effects may include hepatotoxicity, polycythaemia, changes in lipids and worsening sleep apnoea.

Vacuum devices and surgical options. These two treatment options are covered in detail on pages 60–3 and 64–8, respectively.

Key references

Barnes P. Sex therapy and erectile dysfunction. In: Carson CC, Kirby RS, Goldstein I, eds. *Textbook of Erectile Dysfunction*. Oxford: Isis Medical Media, 1999.

Lue TF. Erectile dysfunction. *N Engl J Med* 2000;342:1802–13.

Morales A, Heaton J, Carson C. Andropause: a misnomer for a true clinical entity. *J Urol* 2000;163: 705–12.

4 Pharmacological treatment

Greater understanding of the physiological mechanism of erection and the role of smooth-muscle relaxation led to the concept of the pharmacologically induced erection as a form of treatment for ED. During the early 1980s, it was established that drugs that relax cavernosal smooth muscle and/or reduce adrenergic sympathetic tone to the penile vasculature induce an erection if administered locally in adequate concentrations. The effects of papaverine, which is a powerful smooth-muscle relaxant, were discovered after inadvertent intracavernous injection during a surgical procedure. Similar physiological and clinical observations led to a number of drugs being studied as potential therapeutic agents for ED (Table 4.1).

TABLE 4.1

Drugs with therapeutic potential in ED

Mechanism of action	Drug
Smooth-muscle relaxation	Papaverine
	Nitroglycerine
	Verapamil
	Vasoactive intestinal polypeptide
	Alprostadil
α-adrenoceptor blockade	Phentolamine
	Phenoxybenzamine
	Yohimbine
	Moxisylyte
Phosphodiesterase type 5 inhibition	Sildenafil
	Vardenafil
	Tadalafil
Central nervous system activity	Apomorphine

Oral pharmacological agents

Sildenafil citrate (Viagra®) is a breakthrough therapy in the treatment of ED (Table 4.2). Nitric oxide, the key neurotransmitter involved in relaxation of corpus cavernosal smooth muscle, acts through a second messenger system involving guanylate cyclase. The cGMP produced is normally broken down by a cGMP-specific PDE 5 (see page 13), which exists principally in the corpora cavernosa. Sildenafil is a selective inhibitor of PDE 5 and therefore enhances the normal vasodilatory erectile mechanisms (Figure 4.1).

Sildenafil has been evaluated in controlled clinical trials involving more than 4000 men aged 19–87 years. The mean duration of ED in these men was 5 years and aetiologies were organic, psychogenic or mixed. The agent works in response to natural sexual stimulation to improve erectile function and is thus called an 'enhancer'. Treatment-related improvements in erections were reported by 70–90% of patients receiving sildenafil, versus 10–30% of men receiving placebo. Doses of 50 mg and 100 mg were well tolerated and highly effective in restoring erectile function in flexible-dose studies (Figure 4.2). Study results from more than 550 patients treated for at least 1 year indicate that the

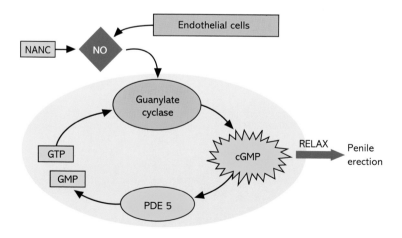

Figure 4.1 Phosphodiesterase type 5 (PDE 5) inhibition prevents cGMP breakdown and thereby enhances the normal erectile response. GTP, guanosine triphosphate; NANC, nonadrenergic–noncholinergic neurones; NO, nitric oxide.

TABLE 4.2

Sildenafil is effective for most cases of ED

- Produces a natural erectile response to sexual stimulation by enhancing the relaxant effect of nitric oxide on the corpora cavernosa
- Effective treatment of ED with broad-spectrum aetiology
- Efficacy is maintained long term
- The therapeutic window is up to 4 hours after administration of a single dose
- Side-effects are predictable, well-tolerated and dose-dependent

efficacy of sildenafil is maintained during long-term treatment (Figure 4.3).

Clinical trial data also demonstrate that sildenafil, taken 1 hour before sexual activity, is effective therapy for ED in a wide variety of patients, including those with diabetes (57%), spinal cord injury (80%), as well as other concomitant medical disorders, such as hypertension (70%) and coronary artery disease (70%). It is also effective in patients taking a wide variety of other medications.

The recommended dose of sildenafil is 50 mg taken approximately 60 minutes before sexual activity; this should be taken no more than once daily. Based on efficacy and tolerance, the dose may be increased

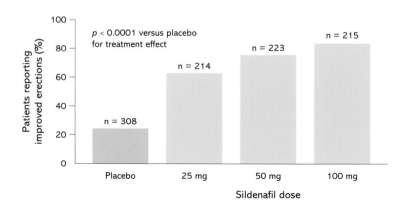

Figure 4.2 Patients treated with sildenafil reported improved erections in clinical trials.

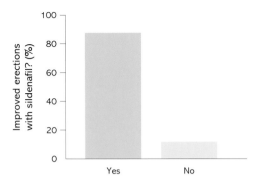

Figure 4.3 After 1 year, most patients still reported improved erections with sildenafil.

to 100 mg or reduced to 25 mg. Optimal response may require as many as 6 to 8 attempts at the most effective dose.

Side-effects and interactions. The adverse events reported in clinical trials with sildenafil were usually transient and mild to moderate in nature. The most commonly reported side-effects were headache (16%), flushing (10%), dyspepsia (7%) and nasal congestion (4%). Altered vision, such as temporary and subtle change in colour or brightness perception, was also reported in a small number of patients; this effect is thought to be due to some inhibitory effect of sildenafil on phosphodiesterase type 6, which is present in the photosensory cells of the retina. No cases of priapism were reported. The overall discontinuation from sildenafil therapy was low – 2.5% compared with 2.3% for those receiving placebo.

Sildenafil is cleared predominantly by cytochrome P450 isozymes in the liver. Cytochrome P450 inhibitors, such as cimetidine, ketoconazole and erythromycin, result in reduced clearance of sildenafil, but this is not usually associated with an increase in adverse events in patients taking this type of medication.

Sildenafil has peripheral vasodilatory properties, resulting in modest decreases in blood pressure in some patients. Consistent with its known effects on the nitric oxide/cGMP pathway, sildenafil is contraindicated in patients using nitrates, such as glyceryl trinitrate and isosorbide, or nitric oxide donors, such as sodium nitroprusside, in any form.

Because of the contraindication of sildenafil in patients using nitrates, concern has arisen about prescribing sildenafil in patients with heart disease. There is currently no evidence of any direct deleterious effect on myocardium. In randomized studies to date, the incidence of significant cardiac events has been the same in both the placebo and sildenafil groups. Sexual intercourse itself is a minor risk factor for myocardial infarction and thus some care must be given before prescribing any treatment that may restore sexual function in an at-risk patient. The exercise involved in sexual intercourse has been equated to walking up two flights of stairs. It is sometimes necessary to confirm with patients that they are capable of this level of exertion. More precise guidelines have been devised for use prior to prescribing any ED treatment in a patient with documented cardiac disease (Table 4.3).

Since the launch of sildenafil in 1998, it has become the first-line treatment of choice for most men presenting with ED. Its high efficacy

TABLE 4.3

Guidelines for prescribing ED treatment in patients with cardiac disease

Risk	Cardiac status	Management
Low	• Controlled hypertension • Mild valvular disease • Mild stable angina • Post re-vascularization	Manage in primary care
Moderate	• Recent MI or cerebrovascular accident (6 weeks) • Congestive heart failure • Murmur of unknown cause • Moderate stable angina	Specialized evaluation recommended
High	• Uncontrolled angina • Uncontrolled hypertension • Severe heart failure • Recent MI or cerebrovascular accident (2 weeks) • High-risk arrhythmia • Hypertrophic cardiomyopathy • Moderate/severe valve disease	Refer for cardiac opinion

and good safety profile have made it the ideal option for both patients and physicians alike. Not everyone is suitable for this drug, however, and the following patient groups need to consider an alternative therapeutic option:

- patients taking any form of nitrate or nitric oxide donor drug
- patients with retinitis pigmentosa
- patients with a very low libido
- patients with significant cardiac disease (see Table 4.3).

Apomorphine (Uprima®, Ixense®). Sexual activity often commences with visual, aural and tactile stimuli (pro-erectile stimuli) acting through higher centres within the brain and the central nervous system. The importance of these central neurohormonal mechanisms to erectile function has made their pathways a target for centrally acting drugs.

Apomorphine is a dopamine-receptor agonist that acts on the dopaminergic receptors in the paraventricular nucleus of the hypothalamus. This area of the brain activates a neural event that coordinates a sequence of signalling that results in a penile erection. The drug therefore acts as a central initiator of an erection by enhancing and coordinating the pro-erectile stimuli.

Apomorphine sublingual (SL) has been administered to more than 3000 men in over 75 000 doses. In the initial phase II placebo-controlled studies, men were administered 2, 4, 5 or 6 mg of apomorphine SL. Results showed a dose–response effect with two-thirds of patients achieving successful intercourse at the highest dose. In phase III crossover double-blind studies, 854 patients were given either apomorphine SL in either 2 or 4 mg doses. The patients were between 18 and 70 years of age, with nearly 75 having moderate or severe ED of multiple aetiologies, and the men had multiple co-morbidities (30% had hypertension, 16% diabetes and 16% coronary artery disease). Outcome measures included intercourse rates and erections firm enough for sexual intercourse as well as partner response evaluations. Erections occurred rapidly (between 10 and 25 minutes). At the higher dose of 4 mg, erections sufficient for intercourse were achieved on 54% of attempts when compared with 33% for placebo. Nausea was the commonest side-effect and was also more common at the higher dose, while syncope was the most significant. There were no serious adverse events.

The drug is marketed at the 2 and 3 mg doses where it provides erections sufficient for intercourse in 45–49% of men (Figure 4.4). At the 2 and 3 mg doses, side-effects were lower than those seen in the original trials where higher doses of the drug were used. The main adverse effects compared with placebo were:

- nausea (7%)
- headache (7%)
- dizziness (4.5%)
- syncope (1%).

No serious adverse events were seen in any of these large clinical trials. Nausea in some patients was most often seen on first dosage of the drug and less commonly seen thereafter. Contraindications are similar to those of the PDE 5 inhibitors and any ED product and include recent myocardial infarction, severe unstable angina and heart failure. Precautions should also be observed in men with uncontrolled hypertension, renal or hepatic failure or those on nitrates or dopaminergic drugs. Patients taking antihypertensive drugs are not affected by co-administration of apomorphine and in a study of 122 men there were no effects on cardiovascular parameters or adverse events.

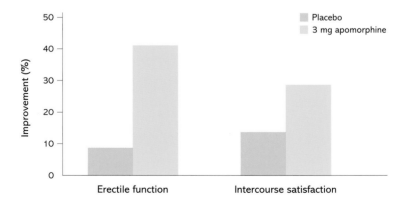

Figure 4.4 Percentage improvement from baseline with apomorphine.

It is expected that apomorphine will become a recognized first-line therapy for men with ED.

Vardenafil is a more biochemically potent phosphodiesterase inhibitor than sildenafil or tadalafil and has undergone phase II and III clinical trials in Europe and North America. Over 1000 men, who have had ED for an average period of 3 years, have been studied in variable-dose placebo-controlled randomized studies. At daily doses of 5, 10 and 20 mg of vardenafil, 77% of men reported improvement in the quality of their erections at the higher dose levels after 12 weeks of treatment, when compared with 28% taking placebo. Similar improvements have been shown for other domains of sexual function such as orgasmic function, intercourse satisfaction and overall satisfaction, with a mean of 70% successfully completed intercourses when taking vardenafil compared with 25% on placebo. Phase III studies on patient sub-groups, such as those with diabetes, have confirmed the safety and efficacy in these men.

Adverse events were those expected of a PDE 5 inhibitor and included headache (13%), flushing (10%), rhinitis (5%) and dyspepsia (6%) at the higher doses, with less frequency at the lower dose. Application for licensing of this drug in the USA has been submitted to the Food and Drug Administration (FDA).

Tadalafil (Cialis™) is another phosphodiesterase inhibitor, which has undergone trials in 4500 subjects. Phase III clinical trials included 1112 patients with a mean age of 59 years and with organic, psychological and mixed etiology with mild, moderate or severe erectile dysfunction. Doses of 5–20 mg were given prior to sexual stimulation and without regard to food intake. Intercourse was successful as early as 16 minutes post-dose in approximately a third of men, and the duration of the therapeutic window of effectiveness was at least 24 hours in 80% of men. These phenomena are due to a rapid tissue distribution and a half-life of 17.5 hours. These characteristics potentially reduce the need for planning associated with most other treatments for erectile dysfunction.

Improved erections were reported in 81% of men taking 20 mg of the drug compared with 35% on placebo. In diabetics the corresponding figure was 76% compared with 32% on placebo. Successful intercourse was possible in 75% of attempts compared with 32% on placebo. The corresponding figure for diabetics was 58% (18% on placebo).

Tadalafil was effective in men taking concomitant medications but, like other PDE 5 inhibitors, is contraindicated in those taking nitrates. Side-effects were mild and transient. There were no serious adverse events attributable to treatment and the discontinuation rate due to adverse events was 1.7% (placebo 1.1%). The most common side-effects for the 10–20-mg dosages were headache (14%), dyspepsia (12%), back pain (6.5%), myalgia (6%) and nasal congestion (4%). Licenses have been applied for in the USA and Europe.

Yohimbine is derived from the bark of the *Pausinystalin yohimbe* tree which, for over a century, has been thought to possess aphrodisiac qualities. Yohimbine has well-defined properties as an α_2-adrenoceptor-blocking agent, acting both peripherally and centrally. In a small study of men with psychogenic impotence, yohimbine has produced a positive response rate of 31% compared with only 5% with placebo; however, in a controlled trial in patients with organic ED, it was found to be no more effective than placebo.

This success has stimulated research into other α_2-blockers with the potential to produce a better response, and drugs with other actions.

Phentolamine is an α-adrenoceptor antagonist that has been used successfully in combination with other agents for intracorporal injection. Experience of its use as a buccal preparation taken 15 minutes prior to intercourse suggested that adequate serum levels for a therapeutic response could be achieved through the oral route of administration. The drug has a dose–response effect in men with ED from all aetiologies, with 53% achieving an erection lasting until ejaculation compared with 38% on placebo. These differences were statistically significant. Side-effects are very similar to those found for yohimbine and other α-blockers, and include tachycardia, hypotension, headache and rhinitis. The side-effect profile has so far precluded regulatory approval of the drug.

Other novel agents. A number of other oral agents are currently under investigation. These include cyclic AMP activators, L-arginine and new nitric oxide donors; of these, L-arginine is the most advanced in terms of clinical trials. Nitric oxide, the key neurotransmitter for erectile function, is synthesized from L-arginine by the enzyme nitric oxide synthetase. It appears that L-arginine may not be effective alone, but may have a role in combination with other oral agents.

Vasoactive drug therapy

Intracavernosal and intraurethral vasoactive drug therapy is often useful in men with ED and particularly effective in men with any form of neurogenic dysfunction. These men have a normal haemodynamic mechanism, but lack the control system that initiates the erectile response; this response can, however, be stimulated by any of the vasoactive agents. This observation is true for any of the neurogenic causes of ED including diabetic autonomic neuropathy. Psychogenic ED, which can also be regarded as a failure of appropriate neurotransmission to the erectile tissues, will often also respond very favourably to this treatment.

As experience with these agents has increased, men with other causes of ED have been treated, in particular men with vascular insufficiency, who form the largest group of patients with organic aetiologies in an ED clinic. High local concentrations of smooth-muscle relaxant drugs act on both the trabecular muscle and the arteriolar vasculature and are able to overcome mild arterial insufficiency. However, when the arterial supply is severely compromised, pharmacologically induced arterial dilatation is ineffective because it cannot facilitate sufficient inflow to engorge the lacunar spaces and thereby operate the veno-occlusive mechanism.

Although all vasoactive drugs produce some degree of erectile response when injected directly into the corpus cavernosum, so far only five have found widespread clinical use: papaverine, phentolamine, prostaglandin E_1, moxisylyte and VIP. The others have failed to do so due to either lack of efficacy or side-effects caused by leakage of the drug into the systemic circulation.

Intracavernosal therapy

The efficacy and safety of self-injection with vasoactive drugs has been demonstrated over the last 10 years. Originally used only by patients with neurogenic impairment, such as spinal cord injuries, this form of treatment has since proved to be effective for men with many other types of erectile disorder (Table 4.4).

Papaverine is a powerful direct smooth-muscle relaxant that acts on both the trabecular muscle of the erectile tissue and the vascular tone, inducing an erection that lasts for several hours. When vasoactive agents were introduced, papaverine was initially the most widely used agent for intracorporal self-injection. It has been extensively studied and shown to be effective. Data from over 4000 men in clinical trials have shown that about 70% of all men who attended an ED clinic obtained an erection sufficient for sexual intercourse. The dose necessary to achieve this can vary from 10 mg to 80 mg, and it is necessary to titrate the dose up to an effective level for each patient to avoid the risk of priapism. For those men who have failed to get an adequate response from papaverine alone, combination therapy with phentolamine and papaverine may prove beneficial. Phentolamine, acting directly on the α-adrenoceptors of the vascular smooth muscle, potentiates the effects of papaverine.

TABLE 4.4

Indications for intracorporal self-injection with vasoactive drugs

Good response
- Psychogenic ED
- Diabetes mellitus
- Neurogenic ED

Moderate response
- Mild arterial insufficiency
- Drug-induced ED
- Mild veno-occlusive disorder
- Age-related ED

Poor response
- Severe arterial insufficiency
- Very elderly men
- Severe veno-occlusive disorder

Phentolamine acts principally to reduce adrenergically induced vascular smooth-muscle tone, and probably does not initiate an erection very effectively on its own. It is used in combination with papaverine and appears to work synergistically with it.

Prostaglandin E$_1$. In 1913, it was established that an extract of human prostate, called prostaglandin, was able to reduce blood pressure. By 1985, prostaglandin E$_1$ was isolated (alprostadil) and had been shown to cause relaxation of smooth muscle in the corpus cavernosum via an adenylate cyclase second messenger system. It is a natural body constituent found in high concentrations in the seminal vesicles and corpora cavernosa, and is actively metabolized in the lung (70% first-pass metabolism), liver and kidney. Alprostadil acts by inhibiting α-adrenergic tone in the penile vasculature and by relaxing trabecular smooth muscle.

Recently, alprostadil has become the drug of choice for intracavernous pharmacotherapy. Prostaglandin E$_1$ plays a natural role as a neurotransmitter in the natural erectile mechanism, and alprostadil is at least as effective in treating ED as combination therapy with papaverine and phentolamine, and appears to have fewer side-effects. As a result, the alprostadil preparations Caverject® and Viridal Duo® have been licensed for the treatment of ED in Europe and the USA. There are now data on over 10 000 men with ED who have undergone self-injection with alprostadil. In one study of 550 men, over 70% of patients achieved an erection sufficient for sexual intercourse that lasted for at least 30 minutes and, in another study, 77% of sexual partners reported the erections to be 'good' or 'very good', with 74% reporting an improvement in their relationship. Studies have demonstrated excellent efficacy in patients failing PDE 5 inhibitor therapy.

The final therapeutic dose of drug must be titrated up to prevent the risk of priapism, although this risk is considerably less than that with papaverine. The effective dose can range from 5 µg to 20 µg depending on the aetiology of the ED. Occasionally, larger doses (up to 60 µg) are required.

Moxisylyte is an α_1-blocker that acts on the sympathetic tone that normally maintains penile flaccidity. Published results suggest that although it appears to have an overall lower efficacy than other injectable agents (46% of patients achieving success in the home), it also has a lower local side-effect profile and is thus well tolerated by patients. Patients with psychogenic causes seem to respond best, though they may require the higher dose of drug (20 mg) to overcome the sympathetic tone. The incidence of side-effects at this higher dose is not increased, with local pain on injection being rare and prolonged erections affecting less than 1%.

Vasoactive intestinal polypeptide is a neurotransmitter that acts on the adenylate cyclase system of the smooth muscle cell, reducing intracellular calcium and initiating relaxation. When used in isolation as an intracavernosal agent, it has a lower efficacy than other injectable agents but has been shown to be very effective in combination with phentolamine (Invicorp™). In a study of over 550 men with predominantly organic ED, 83% were able to achieve erections with one of the two doses available. Adverse events were uncommon, with prolonged erections occurring in only 3 men, and pain on injection was rarely reported. Phentolamine–VIP and the injector device are well tolerated by patients and partners alike. The combination has undergone phase III trials and is awaiting regulatory approval at the time of press.

Combination therapy. In men who fail to get an adequate response from papaverine alone, combination therapy with phentolamine, papaverine and prostaglandin E_1 often proves beneficial. Phentolamine, acting directly on the α-adrenoceptors of the vascular smooth muscle, appears to potentiate the effects of papaverine.

Other vasoactive drugs and drug combinations, such as the combination of phentolamine and VIP, are being introduced and their therapeutic potential is currently under evaluation. The vasoactive agents discussed here can also be used in combination with sildenafil.

Contraindications. Papaverine, phentolamine and alprostadil have a low rate of leakage into the systemic circulation, resulting in few

TABLE 4.5

Relative contraindications to vasoactive drug therapy

- Sickle-cell trait or disease
- Leukaemia
- Anticoagulation
- Poor manual dexterity
- Blood-borne infections, such as HIV or hepatitis
- Previous history of priapism

contraindications to their use. There are, however, some relative contraindications (Table 4.5).

Self-injection technique. Many patients attending an ED clinic will be given a trial injection of a vasoactive drug in an effort not only to establish the possible origin of their problem, but also to test the efficacy of the drug as a potential therapy. If efficacy is proven and the patient wishes to proceed, then he will need to be taught the self-injection technique (Figure 4.5).

The person who demonstrates the technique should administer increasing doses of the vasoactive agent of choice until a good quality erection is obtained. With alprostadil, the recommended starting dose is 1.25 µg for patients with known neurogenic or psychogenic impotence, and 2.5 µg for others, with the dose being doubled on each successive injection. With papaverine, the starting point may be 5 mg, increasing in 5 mg increments. These recommendations are suitable for patients with suspected neurogenic or psychogenic ED, but if there is known arterial insufficiency, the starting dose is usually higher. When a satisfactory erection is achieved, the patient and his partner will gain confidence with the technique.

First, the patient, or his partner, must become familiar with the handling of the needles and syringes and the technique of drawing up drug solutions. In addition, alprostadil needs to be reconstituted from powder prior to injection. The skin over the penis is drawn taut, and the needle and syringe held at right angles to

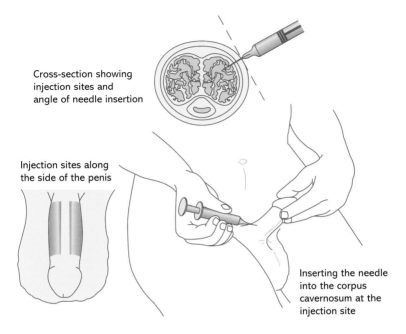

Cross-section showing injection sites and angle of needle insertion

Injection sites along the side of the penis

Inserting the needle into the corpus cavernosum at the injection site

Figure 4.5 Self-injection technique.

the penis (Figure 4.5). The injection is given near to the base of the penis on either side and avoiding any visible veins. Injection sites should be varied. Teaching demonstrations, illustrated manuals and videos, which are all available from the manufacturers, are recommended.

Side-effects from self-injection of vasoactive agents (Table 4.6) can be classified as:

TABLE 4.6

Comparison of side-effects of injectable agents

	Alprostadil (%)	VIP plus phentolamine (%)
Priapism	0.5–1.3	< 0.5
Pain on injection	17–50	1
Haematoma	3	3
Systemic effects	1	10–50

- treatment failure
- unwanted local effects
- unwanted vasodilatory systemic effects (e.g. flushing and hypotension).

Treatment failure. The most common side-effect is treatment failure: 80% of failures are due to incorrect administration of the drug into the corpora cavernosa, usually as a result of incorrect injection technique. If injections continue to be ineffective despite correct technique, a higher drug dose may be necessary. Systemic side-effects are uncommon (about 1%) and result from leakage of the drug into the circulation. Phentolamine has been reported to occasionally cause dizziness, tachycardia and hypotension, as has alprostadil, and papaverine has been associated with occasional derangement of liver function. These observations have not led to any significant limitation in the use of these agents.

Priapism. The most troublesome side-effect with any of these drugs is the development of a prolonged erection, or priapism. Any erection lasting for 4 hours or more, especially if painful, should be regarded as a priapism and treatment should be sought. Patients *must* be warned in advance of this potential complication, both verbally and in writing, and should be given instructions on what they should do in the event of a priapism. The occurrence of priapism is dose-dependent with each of the drugs, and tends to occur during the early stages of titration during a treatment programme. The incidence of priapism after injection with alprostadil has been reported to be between 0.5% and 1.3%.

If a priapism does occur, medical intervention should be sought within 6–8 hours. Failure to achieve detumescence after 6–8 hours can cause irreversible ischaemic damage to the corpora cavernosa with subsequent fibrotic damage and permanent loss of erectile function. In most cases, priapism can be relieved by simple aspiration of blood (in 50–100 ml portions) through an appropriate calibre needle placed in the corpora cavernosa.

Other local side-effects include the formation of fibrotic nodules around the injection site after repeated use (which can lead to penile curvature), haematoma formation, and the presence of diffuse pain along the shaft of the penis immediately after injection. Discomfort in the penile shaft is thought to be more common with the use of alprostadil than the other vasoactive drugs, but this does not often result in the cessation of therapy.

Intraurethral therapy

Alprostadil has been developed for insertion into the urethra as a pellet through a specific polypropylene applicator. Once delivered, the pellet dissolves into the urethral mucosa and from there enters the corpora.

Alprostadil is a synthetic form of prostaglandin E_1; it acts via the adenylate cyclase system to reduce intracellular calcium and induce smooth-muscle relaxation. The system for this administration of alprostadil is marketed as MUSE® (Medicated Urethral System for Erection; Figure 4.6). Before use, men are asked to urinate as this aids insertion of the applicator and facilitates the intraurethral dispersion of the drug. While in the sitting position, the patient inserts the applicator and then depresses the ejector button, releasing the alprostadil pellet. The penis is then held upright and gently rolled to disperse the drug. Erections develop about 10–15 minutes after application and last for approximately 30 minutes.

Early results with this treatment reported a dose–response effect in 66% of men with ED (all causes) obtaining a full erection, though subsequent studies have reported a lower efficacy. The doses required to achieve this ranged from 125 to 1000 μg. The side-effects of this treatment are those of urethral pain (7%) and minor urethral trauma (1%). In a comparative study of intracavernosal and intraurethral application of alprostadil, the intracavernosal administration was shown to be more

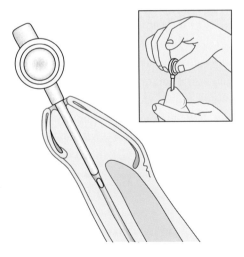

Figure 4.6 Intraurethral administration of alprostadil using the MUSE® system.

effective though there was a slightly higher incidence of local side-effects than with the intraurethral route of administration. It would thus seem that while the intraurethral route of administration is associated with a lower overall success rate, the improved side-effect profile and acceptability to patients may make it a preferred option for some patients. MUSE may also be effective in men with failed penile implants.

Androgen replacement therapy for hypogonadal men

Oral administration. Two types of oral testosterone are available – modified and unmodified. Unmodified testosterone is rapidly absorbed and degraded by the liver, making it difficult to achieve satisfactory serum concentrations. Modified 17-alkyltestosterones, such as methyltestosterone or fluoxy-mesterone, usually require large doses and multiple daily dose regimens. In addition, these compounds are associated with occasional idiosyncratic hepatotoxicity, even at relatively low doses.

Testosterone undecanoate (Andriol®) is an oral testosterone medication available in Canada and Europe. Liver toxicity is significantly reduced because it is absorbed through the lymphatics, and the drug appears to be effective although multiple pills must be taken each day to maintain an adequate serum testosterone level.

Intramuscular injection. Testosterone is esterified for intramuscular administration to prevent rapid degradation and to render it more soluble in oily vehicles (which carry the drug in muscle tissue). Although until recently intramuscular administration was the delivery method of choice, there are a number of significant drawbacks. These include abnormally high initial serum concentrations of testosterone and oestradiol, followed by a decline to subnormal levels before the next injection. Testosterone depot therapy has been reported to produce positive and negative fluctuations in libido, erectile function, energy and mood, in parallel with the variations in serum androgen levels. In addition, patients often find deep intramuscular injections painful and dislike the frequent visits to the doctor that are required.

Testosterone skin patches. Several forms of testosterone skin patch are now approved (Andropatch™ and Virormone™). In hypogonadal men, daily application of testosterone patches produces hormone levels that parallel the endogenous pattern of serum testosterone characteristic of normal men. Patients report improvements in mood, energy, libido and sexual function to a statistically significant greater extent than seen with placebo. The only side-effects are transient local itching, skin irritation and discomfort related to the patch. A new transdermal delivery system (Testoderm™) uses the skin of the scrotum, which allows testosterone to be rapidly absorbed and thus requires only a small patch. The patch adheres gently to the shaved scrotal skin and does not produce skin irritation. Providing the patient has a low free circulating testosterone level, testosterone-replacement therapy can be effective, not only in improving sexual function, but also enhancing well-being and drive.

Pharmacological treatment – Key points

- Sildenafil is effective in approximately 70% of all men with ED, and in these it works in about 70% of attempts at sexual intercourse.
- Sildenafil should not be taken with nitrate drugs but is otherwise well tolerated.
- Apomorphine appears to be slightly less effective than sildenafil but may be faster acting.
- Several new phosphodiesterase inhibitors are undergoing clinical trials and are expected to receive regulatory approval in the near future.
- Prostaglandin E_1 remains the treatment of choice for self-injection therapy.
- Intraurethral therapy is less effective than self-injection therapy but is an alternative for men who fail to respond to oral drug treatment.

Testosterone gel. A 1% testosterone gel (Androgel™) is available in 2.5 g and 5 g doses and has been approved by the FDA in the USA. The gel is applied without a patch once daily and has excellent androgen activity with less skin reactivity than skin patches. Because it is applied once daily, early high levels with subsequent falls in serum testosterone concentrations occur in a diurnal pattern. This medication, which mimics diurnal testosterone production, appears to be more physiological than the intermuscular injection or the oral agents. A new dihydrotestosterone gel is currently undergoing clinical trials and, once approved, this more active form of testosterone may replace other transdermal testosterone preparations.

Alternative medicine therapies

There have been a multitude of therapies devised over the centuries to treat ED. Many of these remedies have become confused with aphrodisiacs, which were aimed at increasing sexual desire rather than ability. Alcohol, herbs, citrus fruit and even the cantharis beetle have variously been described to possess powers that aid ED. In fact, the cantharis beetle contains cantharidinic acid, which can cause an erection but is also nephrotoxic and may lead to priapism and even death. In the last century, monkey testes were transplanted into men to restore erections, and many penile prostheses were devised. The variety of alternative medicines continues to flourish with pheromones, musks, Maca and herbal extracts being readily available. Many of these products contain a number of constituents, some of which contain yohimbine, and therefore some biological activity can be anticipated. The majority, however, have not undergone any form of conventional clinical trial to confirm their safety or efficacy.

Key references

Auerbach S, Agne K, Buttler S et al. Efficacy and safety of escalating doses of 2, 3 and 4 mg apomorphine SL in the treatment of patients with ED. *Int J Impot Res* 2000;(Suppl Nov):22.

Becker AJ, Stief CG, Machtens S et al. Oral phentolamine as treatment for erectile dysfunction. *J Urol* 1998;159: 1214–15.

Boolell M, Gepi-Attee S, Gingell JC, Allen MJ. Sildenafil, a novel effective oral therapy for erectile dysfunction. *Br J Urol* 1996;78:257–61.

Dula E, Nuys V, Buttler S et al. Efficacy and safety of apomorphine SL versus placebo for ED in patients with coronary artery disease. *Int J Impot Res* 2000;(Suppl Nov):23.

Eardley I. New oral therapies for the treatment of erectile dysfunction. *Br J Urol* 1998;81:122–7.

Goldstein I, Lue TF, Padma-Nathan H *et al*. Oral sildenafil in the treatment of erectile dysfunction. *N Engl J Med* 1998; 338:1397–404.

Jackson G, Betteridge J, Dean J et al. A systematic approach to ED in the cardiovascular patient: a consensus statement. *Int J Clin Pract* 1999;53: 445–51.

Lee LM, Stevenson RW, Szasz G. Prostaglandin E1 versus phentolamine papaverine for the treatment of erectile impotence: a double-blind comparison. *J Urol* 1989;141:549–50.

Levine SB, Althof SE, Turner LA et al. Side-effects of self-administration of intracavernous papaverine and phentolamine for the treatment of impotence. *J Urol* 1989;141:54–7.

Linet OI, Ogring FG. Efficacy and safety of intracavernosal alprostadil in men with erectile dysfunction. *N Engl J Med* 1996;334:873–7.

Moncada Iribarren I, Saenz de Tejada I. Pharmacological treatment of erectile dysfunction. *Curr Opin Urol* 1999;9:547–51.

Padma-Nathan H, Giuliano F. Oral drug therapy for erectile dysfunction. *Urol Clin N Am* 2001;28:321–34.

Padma-Nathan H, Hellstrom WJG, Kaiser FE et al. Treatment of men with erectile dysfunction with transurethral alprostadil. *N Engl J Med* 1997;336:1–7.

Porst H, Rosen R, Padma-Nathan H et al. The efficacy and tolerability of vardenafil, a new, oral, selective phosphodiesterase type 5 inhibitor, in patients with erectile dysfunction. *Int J Impot Res* 2001;13:192–9.

Porst H. Transurethral alprostadil with MUSE vs intracavernous alprostadil – a comparative study in 103 patients with erectile dysfunction. *Int J Impot Res* 1997;9:187–92.

Rendell M, Rajfer J, Wicker PA. Sildenafil for treatment of ED in men with diabetes. *JAMA* 1999;281:421–6.

Stakl W, Hasun R, Marberger M. Prostaglandin E1 in the treatment of erectile dysfunction. *World J Urol* 1990;8:84–6.

Virag R. Intracavernous injection of papaverine for erectile failure. *Lancet* 1982;ii:938.

The vacuum constriction device is one of the most time-honoured methods of treating ED. Its design was first patented in 1917 by Dr Otto Lederer and, although the construction and design of the devices has become more sophisticated, the concept remains the same – a vacuum is applied to the penis for a few minutes, causing tumescence and rigidity, which is sustained using a constricting ring at the base of the penis.

Physiology

The physiological changes that occur in a penis during a vacuum-induced erection are quite different from those that occur during a normal or even a pharmacologically induced erection. Trabecular smooth-muscle relaxation does not occur; blood is simply trapped in both the intracorporal and extracorporal compartments of the penis. Distal to the constricting band of the device, venous stasis and decreased arterial inflow lead to penile distension, but also to cyanosis, oedema and a progressive drop in skin temperature. Consequently, vacuum-induced erections eventually become uncomfortable and should not be maintained for more than 30 minutes. In addition, the penis only becomes rigid distal to the constricting bands, rather than along the whole corporal length. As a result, the penis tends to pivot inconveniently at its base.

Equipment and technique

Although many different devices are now manufactured, they all have three common components: a vacuum chamber, a pump and a constriction band that is applied to the base of the penis once an erection is achieved (Figure 5.1). The vacuum chamber is made of clear plastic and is open at one end. This is placed over the penis and, with the help of a lubricant jelly, a seal is formed between the chamber and skin, and the pump mechanism then creates a vacuum of at least 100 mmHg, which draws in sufficient blood to create an erection.

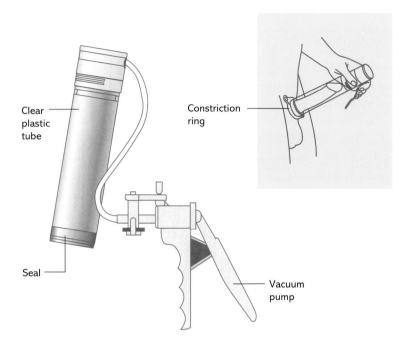

Clear plastic tube

Constriction ring

Seal

Vacuum pump

Figure 5.1 A typical vacuum erection device which is placed over the penis and used to induce an erection that is maintained with a constriction ring.

The pump mechanism may be either attached to the vacuum chamber itself or separate from it, and may be either hand or battery operated. Once an erection develops, an elastic ring (the constriction band) slips off the chamber and maintains the rigidity by preventing blood escape without injury to the penis. These constriction rings are available in a variety of different sizes.

Clinical use

Because the mechanism of erection is non-physiological, the vacuum constriction device is theoretically suitable for most men who experience ED. Indeed, in one study, 98% of men were able to achieve an erection sufficient for sexual intercourse using one of these devices. In clinical practice, the proportion of men who successfully use this technique is about the same as that who find satisfaction with intracavernosal self-injection. In one report, men who responded well to papaverine were the same group of men who responded well to the vacuum device. As with self-injection, there are some instances when caution should be observed (Table 5.1).

Side-effects

Complications arising from the use of these devices are generally of a minor nature. Petechiae due to capillary rupture are common and transient (10%); haematoma formation is less common (about 5% of patients) and often associated with application of a vacuum pressure that is too high. Other complaints from men using these devices include numbness in the penis (occurring in 75% of users at some stage), a feeling of cold, blue discoloration of the penis and altered or diminished sensation of orgasm (Table 5.2). Orgasm is often dry, due to the constriction ring which compresses the urethra and so prevents normal ejaculation and often causes some discomfort. Users have also commented on the lack of spontaneity of sexual relations associated with the use of these devices. Despite these complaints, some men do

TABLE 5.1

Relative contraindications to the use of vacuum devices

- Sickle-cell trait or disease
- Leukaemia
- Anticoagulation, bleeding disorders
- Poor manual dexterity

TABLE 5.2

Side-effects of vacuum devices

Numbness/penis feels cold	75%
Lack of ejaculation	50%
Altered sensation at orgasm	25%
Haematoma/petechiae formation	15%
Discomfort on orgasm	9–11%

> **Vacuum devices – Key points**
>
> - A vacuum erection device (VED) is an effective treatment option for most aetiologies of ED.
> - The side-effects are prohibitive for some men.
> - The treatment does not involve the use of any drugs.

not seem to be deterred from using vacuum devices and most studies show a reasonable rate of patient and partner satisfaction (68–83%) with the technique.

Key references

Bodansky HJ. Treatment of erectile dysfunction using active vacuum assist devices. *Diabetic Med* 1994;11:410–12.

Bosshardt RJ, Farwerk R, Sikora R et al. Objective measurement of the effectiveness, therapeutic success and dynamic mechanisms of the vacuum device. *Br J Urol* 1995;75:786–91.

Nadig PW. Vacuum erection devices. A review. *World J Urol* 1990;8: 114–17.

Wespes E, Schulman CC. Haemodynamic study of the effect of vacuum device on human erection. *Int J Impot Res* 1990;2:337.

Surgical treatment of ED is usually reserved for patients in whom more conservative therapy has failed, or for whom conservative therapy is contraindicated. Most of these patients will have significant arterial or venous disease, penile corpus cavernosum fibrosis, or will, by choice, prefer the prospect of a 'one-off' solution. While the outcome of surgical intervention may be more reliable in certain selected patients, the incidence of morbidity and complications is significantly greater than with medical treatment.

Penile prosthetic implants

Surgically implantable penile prostheses are classified as either semi-rigid or inflatable. Many types with various modifications are widely available. Implants provide penile rigidity and erectile size that adequately simulate the normal physiological erectile state required for sexual intercourse. After careful assessment and discussion with the patient and his partner on their preference, the implants are sized during surgery. The degree of flaccidity differs according to the type of device selected.

Semi-rigid rod prostheses

Semi-rigid rod devices were the first prostheses designed to restore erections and erectile function, and are still used extensively. A variety of semi-rigid rod penile prostheses of different designs are currently available. These prostheses consist of two flexible rods or cylinders that can be varied in length by trimming the proximal portion or adding measured extensions to the proximal portion to fit the patient's measurements (Figure 6.1). Curvature is adjusted via the flexibility provided in their design which usually includes a central, braided metal wire allowing upward or downward deviation of the prosthesis. Mechanical modifications of these devices include hinges to increase the flexibility and ability to position the prosthesis.

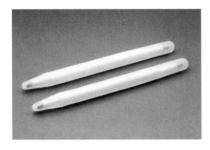

Figure 6.1 Semi-rigid rod penile prostheses are implanted into the corpora cavernosa. They comprise two rods that are trimmed in length intra-operatively, fitted in width, and adjusted in curvature through the flexibility provided in their design.

Surgical implantation of these semi-rigid rod prostheses is the simplest type of procedure. A dorsal, subcoronal penile incision, a penoscrotal incision, ventral penile incision, or a perineal incision may be used to access the corpora cavernosa for dilatation of the corpora and implantation.

Inflatable penile prostheses
Inflatable penile prostheses are available in self-contained, two-piece, and three-piece designs (Figures 6.2 and 6.3).

Two-piece inflatable penile prostheses contain two completely inflatable cylinders and a pump/reservoir. This pump/reservoir provides a limited, but usually adequate, volume of fluid for inflation and deflation of the prosthesis. The two-piece design avoids the need for an abdominal fluid reservoir, which is used in three-piece inflatable prostheses. The two-piece design also has an advantage over the self-contained prostheses by increasing the volume of fluid placed in the penile cylinders to improve both erectile inflation and flaccidity. Because of the size of the pump/reservoir, however, flaccidity may not be as complete as with the three-piece inflatable prostheses. Implantation of this device is similar to that described below for the three-piece inflatable penile prosthesis.

Three-piece inflatable penile prostheses are the most complex, yet most cosmetic penile prosthetic devices available. Two inflatable cylinders are placed in the hollow corpora cavernosa and connected to a small pump device placed in the scrotum lateral to the testicle, which is used to inflate and deflate the cylinders, thereby simulating a normal erection.

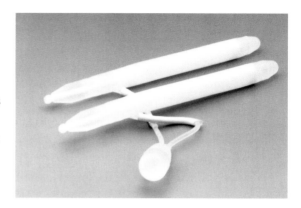

Figure 6.2
A two-piece inflatable prosthesis with a combined pump and reservoir.

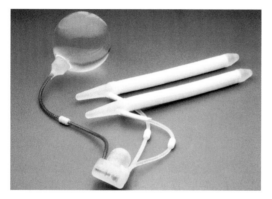

Figure 6.3
A three-piece inflatable implant showing the separate pump, reservoir and cylinders.

Saline is provided from a reservoir placed beneath the rectus muscles of the abdomen. Because of the significant volume provided by this reservoir for both inflation and deflation, both the erect and flaccid states produced are usually excellent. The three-piece inflatable prosthesis provides increased girth and length in comparison to other devices and the more natural flaccid state facilitates the positioning and carriage of the prosthesis under clothing.

Postoperative care

An ice pack may be applied to the genitalia after the operation, and patients are treated with antibiotics to prevent infection. Oral analgesics are also administered. In addition, with inflatable devices, patients are asked to check the position of the pump for 4–6 weeks before activation to maintain its dependent position in the scrotum. Patients

> **Surgical treatment – Key points**
>
> - Surgery involves dilatation of the erectile tissue of the penis and therefore is a last resort of treatment.
> - Penile prostheses have an incidence of infection at insertion and a mechanical failure rate.
> - Satisfactory results, for patient and partner alike, can be achieved when other treatments have failed.

are then asked to return to learn how to activate and deflate the device 6 weeks or so after the operation.

Postoperative complications. Although the incidence of postoperative complications has decreased markedly over the past decade, mechanical malfunction can still occur with any of the penile prosthetic devices. The semi-rigid rod penile prostheses may require replacement due to cable fracture, or reduced rigidity. Inflatable prostheses are, however, more likely to suffer mechanical complications, although reported mechanical malfunction rates are currently less than 5% over 3 years. Fluid leakage is the most common problem with inflatable prostheses; fluid leaks most commonly occur in the cylinders, which are the portion of the device under the highest pressure. In all cases, device malfunction requires surgical exploration and replacement of the faulty parts of the prosthesis.

Another potential complication is infection; this occurs in 3–5% of patients with penile prostheses. Higher infection rates can be expected in patients who have had alterations or repairs to their prosthesis, and those with autoimmune diseases and diabetes mellitus. Prosthesis removal, healing, and subsequent replacement is the usual procedure for patients with infection. Other complications that can arise include erosion of the prosthesis, sustained pain, reduced penile length and reduction in sensation. These complications, though rare, are of significant concern to those men affected and their partners, as well as the surgeon involved.

Patient and partner satisfaction

A number of studies have assessed the outcome and the degree of postoperative satisfaction of patients undergoing penile prosthesis implantation. In general, satisfaction rates are high with all types of implant. The success of surgical treatment is linked to expectations as well as the relationship between the patient and his partner, and the psychological state of the patient preoperatively. One study comparing satisfaction rates identified no significant difference in patient satisfaction with the semi-rigid and inflatable devices, but when the patients' sexual partners were included in the survey, increased satisfaction with inflatable implants was noted.

Key references

Beutler LE, Scott FB, Karacan I et al. Women's satisfaction with partner's penile implant: inflatable versus noninflatable prosthesis. *Urology* 1984;24:552–8.

Carson CC. Penile prostheses. In: Carson CC, Kirby RS, Goldstein I, eds. *Textbook of Erectile Dysfunction*. Oxford: Isis Medical Media, 1999.

Carson CC, Mulcahy JJ, Govier FE. Efficacy, safety and patient satisfaction outcomes of the AMS 700 CX inflatable penile prosthesis: results of a long-term, multicenter study. *J Urol* 2000;164:628–33.

Steege JF, Stout AL, Carson CC. Patient satisfaction in Scott and Small-Carrion penile implant recipients: a study of 52 patients. *Arch Sex Behav* 1986;15:393–9.

Woodworth BE, Carson CC, Webster GD. Inflatable penile prosthesis: effect of device modification on function longevity. *Urology* 1991;38:533–6.

A number of medical conditions are commonly associated with ED, including:
- depression
- diabetes mellitus
- hypertension
- vascular disease
- endocrine abnormalities.

Other situations and conditions are associated with ED, though the link is not recognized. Awareness of them should mean patients can be warned of the risk of ED, and early diagnosis and treatment can occur.

Peyronie's disease

Peyronie's disease is curvature of the penis due to fibrosis within the tunica albuginea. The affected corpora cavernosa cannot lengthen on erection, leading to curvature. The condition is most common in middle-aged men who are sexually active. Its exact aetiology remains unknown, but it may result from trauma and bleeding into the tunica, followed by activation of the inflammatory process and fibrosis. The more recent observation that HLA class II antigens are more common in men with Peyronie's disease suggests an underlying autoimmune cause. Erectile dysfunction occurs in 30–40% of men with Peyronie's disease. Although the mechanism of their ED is not clearly understood, most appear to have a vascular problem, such as arterial insufficiency where the fibrosis actually distorts the vessels, or failure of the veno-occlusive mechanism.

To a certain extent, treatment is determined by whether the patient has ED and Peyronie's disease. If the patient has this combination, he may be best advised to undergo insertion of a penile implant, as surgical straightening of the penis alone is unlikely to overcome the ED. If penile curvature alone is the factor that precludes intercourse, surgical correction of the curvature by plaque excision and grafting or the Nesbit operation is favoured. This latter procedure involves shortening of the contralateral corpus cavernosum. Patients should be warned of the risks of penile shortening and onset of ED after surgery.

Renal failure

Chronic renal impairment is associated with a high incidence of ED, with the incidence increasing with the level of creatinine. Erectile dysfunction is present in about 50% of patients by the time they require dialysis. A number of factors may be involved, including:

- anaemia
- autonomic neuropathy
- reduced testosterone levels with elevated prolactin
- accelerated arterial disease
- other drug therapies
- psychological stress.

After successful transplantation and normalization of renal function, erectile function is restored in many patients. Erythropoietin treatment in patients with renal impairment can also improve the patient's overall quality of life and erectile function.

Pelvic surgery

Any form of pelvic surgery can lead to nerve damage affecting the erectile mechanism. The cavernous nerves run from the pelvic plexus on the lateral border of the rectum down postero-lateral to the prostate and into the base of the penis. Damage is, therefore, most likely to occur following surgery to the rectum, bladder or prostate. Improved knowledge of the anatomical course of these nerves has led to the development of surgical techniques, aided by the Cavermap® nerve stimulation apparatus, that aim to preserve them where possible, but damage cannot be avoided during some operations for malignant disease.

Patients who undergo gastrointestinal surgery that results in an ileostomy or colostomy may suffer depression or loss of self-esteem, which may cause ED. This is particularly relevant to sufferers of inflammatory bowel disease requiring excision of the rectum and ileostomy. Patients should always be made aware that specific surgical procedures may lead to ED (Table 7.1). Preliminary evidence suggests

TABLE 7.1

Risks of ED associated with surgery

Procedure	Reported risks (%)
Radical prostatectomy	10–90
Radical cystectomy	50–90
Transurethral resection of the prostate	8
Anterior resection of rectum	10–50

that the sooner pharmacological treatment is started after an operation, the more likely the patient is to regain normal erectile function.

Penile injuries

Damage to either the corpora cavernosa or to the neurovascular bundles that supply the corpora can lead to failure of the erectile mechanism. Recently, it has been suggested that prolonged cycling may cause traumatic injury to the pudendal nerves, presumably due to neurovascular compression from the saddle.

Corporal injuries

Blunt or penetrating injuries can cause rupture of the tunica albuginea. If not surgically repaired immediately, such injuries can lead to persistent venous leakage through the defect, causing failure of normal corporal filling. The most common cause of blunt trauma is penile fracture (i.e. rupture of the tunica albuginea). This may occur during sexual intercourse or masturbation, and is characterized by an audible crack, followed by penile pain, loss of erection and the onset of a penile haematoma.

Treatment involves urgent exploration and repair of the corporal defect, which should preserve potency in most cases. If repair is delayed for 36 hours or more, ED or penile deformity on erection is a likely consequence.

Neurovascular bundle injuries

Urethral trauma is the most common cause of injury to the neurovascular bundle, after surgery. It may occur either after a perineal injury and bulbar urethral damage or a pelvic fracture injury and membranous urethral damage. In either instance, it is the neurovascular bundle running posterolateral to the apex of the prostate and posterior urethra that is disrupted. The further the injury is away from the membranous urethra, the less likely it is that ED will result. Thus anterior urethral trauma only occasionally results in this problem.

Complete urethral disruption injuries from a pelvic fracture are almost universally associated with ED, which may be difficult to treat. Patients often have a combination of both neurological and vascular impairment. Consequently, they do not often respond to conventional pharmacological treatments. In some cases, arterial revascularization surgery should be considered, as this is the subgroup of patients most likely to benefit.

Useful addresses

Doctors

www.nlm.nih.gov
The website of the National Library of Medicine (USA) has descriptions of the causes and treatments of ED as well as some of the latest literature from the medical press.

www.afud.org
The American Foundation for Urological Disease website provides a comprehensive survey of all forms of urological conditions including the causes and management of ED.

www.medicinenet.com
A comprehensive medical directory of all forms of medical conditions with clear descriptions of ED and the treatment options available.

www.informed.org.uk
A website about general medical conditions with reviews of current aspects of causes, diagnosis and treatment of ED.

www.esir.net
This site provides both a regular newsletter and current scientific information on latest research into products and drugs related to ED.

www.erectilefunction.org

Patients

www.informed.org.uk
A website about general medical conditions with reviews of current aspects of causes, diagnosis and treatment of ED.

www.impotence.org.uk
Contains information about different forms of sexual dysfunction, patient information leaflets about these and several sexual problems including premature ejaculation, gay sex and ED.

www.medicinenet.com
A comprehensive medical directory of medical conditions with clear descriptions of the causes and treatments of ED.

www.iiem.org
A coalition website of several international organizations involved in the care of men with ED.

www.esir.net
This site provides a patient guide through the diagnosis and management of ED as well as a newsletter with current news and information.

www.embarrassingproblems.com
Provides information and advice on a wide range of problems which many people find too embarassing to discuss with a physician.

Index